Almond Oil for Health and Beauty

Discover the Various Health, Beauty and Culinary Secrets of This

Vitamin Rich Oil

Disclaimer

Summary

Almond contains 44% of oil, which is rich in nutrients and this is the reason why it has been used for ages for various purposes. Normally when we think of oils, we think of cooking. But that's not the case with almond oil. Besides cooking, it is used for a lot of other purposes which we will further discuss in this e-Book.

Here you can learn about almond oil's use for

1. Skin

2. Hair

3. Massage therapies

4. Soaps and cosmetics

5. Cooking

And so much more!

If you want to know about several other benefits of almond oil, then you need to read ahead!

Contents

Almond Oil – Extraction and Characteristics

Different methods are used to extract almond oil: there are industrial ones that are used for mass production of almond oil and there are others that are used for the production of oil on a smaller scale. The most common method used for this purpose is cold pressing that obtains oil from dried almonds. This method can be used for home production of almond oil as well.

Making Almond Oil At Home

This method does not require any special industrial equipment; just a simple blender or manually operated oil press would suffice. Follow these steps and you can easily prepare almond oil at your home.

1. **What you need?** – All you need is 3 teaspoons of olive oil and 2 cups of almonds; and of course, a blender. If you are using an oil press then you need to toast the almonds before starting the preparation process.

2. **Blending** – Next, blend both ingredients; gradually taking the blender from low speed to high speed.

3. **Solid alm**onds – After some time you will see solid pieces of almond turning into small balls and depositing at the walls of the blender. Remove these solid pieces from the side of the blender and deposit them in the center, then continue blending.

4. **Add olive oil** – Now start adding olive oil in the blender, one teaspoon at a time. It will speed up the blending process.

5. **Oil** – The constant blending will gradually increase the consistency of the blender mixture and you will get nut meat. Transfer this nut meat in an airtight jar and keep it in the refrigerator. After a few days, the nut meat will start releasing oil. This oil can be used for one of the various purposes mentioned below.

Characteristics of Almond Oil

1. Almond oil contains linoleic and oleic acid, which are essential fatty acids that enhance metabolism.

2. This oil is rich in various types of minerals (calcium, magnesium, iron, manganese, zinc and selenium), vitamins (B-complex group and vitamin E) and dietary fiber.

3. Almond oil is gluten free, making it ideal cooking oil for patients with celiac disease and gluten allergies.

4. There are basically two varieties of almond oil: these are sweet almond oil and of course, almond oil. Normal almond oil is made of roasted almonds and you can detect the flavor of almonds in them. On the contrary, you cannot detect the flavor of almonds in sweet almond oil.

Skin Care

There are various ways in which almond oil can help you maintain your skin.

Healthy Skin

As mentioned above, almond oil is rich in minerals and vitamins that is why its external application can do miracles for your skin. The best thing about this oil is that it is compatible for all skin types. Whether you have oily skin or dry skin, it won't cause your skin any harm unlike other chemical products that are designed for certain skin types only.

Skin pores easily absorb almond oil; therefore, you don't have to worry about accumulation of dust particles in the pores of your skin, which is a very common problem with people who have oily skin and often leads to acne problems. Moreover, the presence of nutrients in the oil acts as an external healing source and enhances the quality of skin; especially for dry skins.

Revitalizes Skin

Oils are generally considered good as moisturizers but almond oil is known for its exfoliation property as well. It cleans the skin by scrubbing off dead skin cells and impurities.

If you don't rely on industrially manufactures scrubs or exfoliators, then you can prepare your almond oil scrub at home by mixing 1 tablespoon of almond oil with 1 teaspoon of sugar. Once you have prepared the mixture, apply it on your face by gently rubbing it in small circles like you would do with other scrubs.

If you use this homemade scrub once every two weeks on your skin, regularly, you will notice a significant change in just a few weeks. Not only will you find a significant glow in your skin, but you will also observe reduction in blackheads, white heads and acne. And the best part is that it is one of the most cost effective scrubbing methods available with no side effects.

Delays Aging

One of the most common aging problems that both men and women are concerned about is wrinkles and skin aging signs. There are several anti aging creams and lotions available that claim to reduce the aging effects in short amount of time but their effects are usually short term and some of them have devastating side effects too.

There is one safe solution available in the form of almond oil. Its anti aging effects are long term but they require equally long time to take effect. So, in short the sooner you start using almond oil on your skin, the longer you can experience its miraculous anti-wrinkling effects; as it fulfills all your nutritional requirements and makes your skin healthy internally as well as externally.

Tip: Here is one of the easiest anti-wrinkling formulas that you prepare at home to reduce the aging effects on your skin. Take two walnuts, crush their insides and mix them with a teaspoon of almond oil and two tablespoon of yogurt. Apply it on your skin gently and when it dries off, remove it by rubbing it off your skin. Use it once a week to get long lasting effects.

An Effective Solution for Eczema and Psoriasis

Almond oil is often used for treating skin problems because it has a soothing effect and reduces inflammation. Psoriasis is a chronic skin disorder that causes inflammation ad constant itching on the skin. Application of almond oil on the effected patches of the skin can reduce the irritation on the skin. Same is the case with eczema.

You need to remember that almond oil does not treat these ailments; it works as an external medicine, one of the most cost effective ones that reduce itching and speeds up the healing process.

Tip: If you are having trouble with eczema, psoriasis or any skin diseases that cause inflammation or itchiness you can prepare this external applicator and apply it on your skin from time to time. Combine 2, 3 drops of vitamin E oil with 2 tablespoons of almond oil, 4 drops of true Lavender essential oil and 4 drops of German Chamomile oil and store it in a jar for further use.

Reduces Acne, Whiteheads and Blackheads

If you have zits, pimples or acne on your skin and you have subjected your skin to several skin products to treat them then you must know that majority of these works as long as you are applying them on your skin. Soon after quitting their application, you will observe that your skin problems have started resurfacing again.

One easy way to treat skin problems is by creating home remedial cures that include almond oil. The reason why you should prefer almond oil over industrially manufactured products is because it has a wide range of nutrients that provide nourishment to the skin which keeps it healthy in the long term and prevents itself from common skin diseases.

Tip: Prepare a skin mask by mixing almond oil, glycerin and lemon juice in equal quantity and apply it on the skin areas that have blackheads and whiteheads. When the mask dries off, remove it gently by rubbing it off the skin. This is the safest and most effective method to remove blackheads and whiteheads.

Protection from Sun

We know that exposure to sunlight means exposure to vitamin D, which is good for the skin but extensive exposure can result in a lot of skin problems like wrinkling, sun burn or rapid aging of skin. Sun blocks and sunscreens reduce the negative effects of sun's UV rays to the minimum. If you are not fond of using chemically enhanced products on your skin then you can always use almond oil.

Journal of Cosmetic Dermatology published in its 2007' issue that application of almond oil not only protects skin against these damaging effects but also treats the problems that were caused due to previous unprotected exposure to sunlight.

Tip: You can prepare sunscreen at your home by mixing the following ingredients: quarter cup of coconut oil, half cup of almond oil, 2 tablespoon of zinc oxide and quarter cup of beeswax. It can be stored up to six months after that you will have to prepare a fresh batch.

Hair Care

A Good Conditioner Substitute

Conditioners are used to add shining to the hair, especially dry hair require conditioning at least once a week. General conditioners available in the market are designed for certain hair types. Not every type of conditioner suits all hair types; therefore, if you are looking for a better alternative, almond oil is what you need! It has a light texture that serves as an ideal substitute for conditioners and can add shine to the hair. You'd be amazed to see that almond oil serves as a better substitute than several other conditioners present in the market.

Tip: Mix almond oil and in water in equal quantity and store it in a spray bottle. You can spray your hair with this oil when they require conditioning, after shampooing. Then lightly massage your scalp with your fingertips so that the oil absorbs. You will notice obvious shine in your hair.

Improves Hair Quality

Hair, like every other part of the body, needs nutrients and proper conditioning and this is why external care is as much important as internal care. The presence of a wide range of nutrients in the almond oil improves hair quality and texture. If you get into the habit of massaging your hair regularly with almond oil, you will notice a considerable difference in the health, strength and outlook of your hair. This is because the massaging enhances the blood circulation in the scalp, and the vitamins and minerals present in the oil fastens the hair repair process and prevents them from falling off.

Once you are done with massaging your scalp with almond oil, take a towel soaked in warm water and wrap it around your hair. This will make sure that the oil gets absorbed properly and doesn't block the pores, which is what actually causes hair fall.

Reduces Hair Fall and Split Ends

Split ends and hair falling is an indication of weak hair. When hairs suffer from deficiency of nutrients, they are subjected to common hair problems. The easiest and the most effective way to deal with these problems is to do oiling every once a week or so and eat healthy food, which means avoiding junk food as much as you can.

Tip: Here is an easy home remedy to reduce split ends and hair fall problems. Combine olive oil, almond oil and castor oil in equal proportions and massage your scalp with this oil mixture. Don't use this too frequently or it can have a negative effect on your hair. Apply this oil mixture once in every few days and after a few days you will notice that your hair problems have reduced considerably.

Reduces Dandruff

Dandruff is generally considered a scalp problem, not a hair problem. Especially people who have dry skin suffer from this problem. However, the methods used to reduce this problem require oiling and oil based stuff to induce moisture in the scalp. You must have seen a lot of chemical products in the market that claim to reduce dandruff in just a few days but one should avoid these products as their effects are short term. You will experience the return of dandruff in your hair right after you stop using these products.

Tip: Mix four tablespoons of yogurt with one tablespoon of almond oil. Apply this yogurt mixture to your hair, making sure that it reaches your scalp. Fold your hair in a bun and let it stand for about half hour; after that, thoroughly wash your hair with shampoo. You can apply this mask once in a month. It can treat dandruff problems and itchiness of the scalp.

Makes Hair Soft

Not only women but men also like to have shiny, soft hair. If scalp gets proper internal and external nourishment, your hair will automatically turn soft and healthy. If you massage your hair regularly with oil and keep your body hydrated, you won't suffer with dry hair issues. But if you can't do that then oiling as frequently as possible and applying hair masks can make your hair soft and shiny.

Tip: Mash one avocado and mix it with almond oil. Apply the mixture to your hair and massage thoroughly. Leave it for half an hour and after that wash your hair with shampoo. Using it once in every two weeks will make your hair soft.

Beauty Benefits

Strong Nails

You don't need expensive nail treatments and cuticle removers to make your nails strong and sturdy; you have a cost effective solution in the form of almond oil. This is one of those treatments that is easily available and have no side effects. Plus, it keeps nails moist and hydrated, which prevents breaking due to drying. So women who want to keep long nails and can't do so because their nails won't grow, almond oil can solve your problems.

Tip: Heat some almond oil in a bowl and when it cools off a bit, soak your nails in it for 5 to 10 minutes. Your nails will get shiny and strong.

Treats Cracked Lips

Dry air, sunlight exposure and cold weather causes chapped lips and unfortunately these are the conditions that you cannot avoid, you can only treat them with proper care. The easiest way to treat cracked or chapped lips is by restoring moisture in them.

You can make your own lip balm using almond oil and use it to treat chapped lips. Mix five drops of almond oil in one tablespoon of honey and store it in a small container. You can use this lip balm whenever you have dry or cracked lips.

Makeup Remover

Almost everyone knows that makeup can damage skin; therefore, one simple way to counteract the negative effects of makeup is by removing it with almond oil. It will clear your skin of all the chemicals and will give you the added advantage of treating it with vitamins and minerals. In addition to that, if you have pimples, acne or skin allergy then almond oil is the safest makeup remover for you. Chemically induced makeup removers can cause more damage to such skin types that can result in a negative reaction.

Tip: Mix almond milk and almond oil in equal quantity, soak a cotton ball in the mixture and use it to clean off your makeup. The enzymes present in the mixture will release the dirt and make it easier for you to clean it off. Plus, it will keep your skin healthy and soft in the long term.

Hand and Foot Care

Cracked feet and dry hands are a common problem in winter but if you massage your hands and feet regularly, you skin won't suffer any damage. Most hand and foot creams make skin greasy, which in turn attracts dust and captures it on the skin. Therefore, in order to keep it clean and un-cracked you need to use a moisturizer that gets easily absorbed in the skin and almond oil fits this criterion perfectly.

Almond oil has a light texture which allows it to get easily absorbed in the skin and it has a sweet fragrance which makes its application on the skin bearable. Moreover, the presence of zinc in this oil speeds up the healing process so if you have cracked heels or dry skin, regular application of almond oil will heal it in just a few days. As soon as your skin mends, you will observe a significant difference in the complexion and health of the skin.

Tip: You can use almond oil to make your own foot lotion at home by mixing a tablespoon of almond oil, olive oil and wheat germ oil each with 12 drops of eucalyptus essentials. Store this mixture in a bottle and massage your feet every night with it.

Good for Eyelashes

Eyelashes may be a small feature of the face but they're not insignificant. Long eyelashes will not only enhance the beauty of your eyes but will make your whole face look stunning. Almond oil is one of those cost effective beauty products that is easily available and promotes the growth of eyelashes.

So, if you are not afraid to have flaunting, to-die-for eyelashes then you should start using almond oil regularly. But wait; don't pour it in your eyes! Keep it in a small bottle on your beauty stand, dip your old mascara brush it in every night and apply it on your eyes as you would apply mascara. One coating should suffice. If you overuse it, it might drip down inside your eyes and cause itching. So, you have to be a bit cautious during its application!

Removes Dark Circles

Late night study sessions, movies nights and all night parties can cause dark circles and damage your whole look. There are several beauty products available in the market that claim to remove dark circles under the eyes in record time but like majority other products their effects last as long as you apply them on the affected area. However, that is not the case with almond oil. The main reason behind this is that it comprises of natural nutrients that have a long lasting effect.

Almond oil's anti aging properties remove puffiness and dark circles under the eyes and it is better than most of the expensive beauty creams available in the market. Its miraculous effects will not be evident right after its first application but after applying it regularly for a few days you will see that the dark circles have started diminishing.

Tip: Before going to sleep, dip your finger tips in almond oil and apply it on the area under your eyes by massaging gently without applying pressure.

Health Benefits

Makes Immunity System Effective

Intake of almond oil is as beneficial as its external application. It strengthens the body from the inside by improving the immunity system. If taken in moderate quantity daily, this oil can help your body in fighting against fever, cold, flu and other common problems. In addition to that, almond oil is one of the best laxatives available! People who take a lot of medicines to treat their digestion problems can let go of them and rely on almond oil to treat these problems.

When taking medicines, one is always conscious about its side effects but with almond oil you don't need to worry about these problems as the presence of vitamins and minerals guarantees no side effects. However, if you consume it in excessive amounts you might suffer negative reactions due to over consumption.

Protects Against Heart Diseases

Heart diseases are usually a result of high consumption and storage of processed fat; on the contrary, consumption of mono-saturated fat can reduce the risk of heart diseases in a person. This is where almond oil steps in!

It is one of those sources that comprises of health promoting fats in addition to folic acid and potassium all of which are known to reduce risk of heart diseases in people. Research studies from 5 different institutes have proven that almond oil's regular consumption can reduce the risk of heart diseases by 30%.

Tip: Replace your regular cooking oil with almond oil and you will feel start feeling the difference in your health in just a few days.

Maintains Blood Cholesterol and Blood Pressure Levels

High blood pressure is a common problem in several people these days, which requires substitution of high sodium ingredients with low sodium ones. Almond oil in one of those ingredients that contains low sodium and high potassium which keeps the blood pressure levels under control.

Moreover, the presence of mono-saturated fats and vitamin E in this oil regulates the blood cholesterol levels as well, reducing the risk of heart diseases. Almonds have LDL lowering effect that reduces the damaging effects of cholesterol from 8% to 12%. LDL is a type of cholesterol that is related with heart diseases and atherosclerosis. All these benefits can be availed by replacing your regular cooking oil with almond oil.

Diminishes Stretch Marks

These days the most common method to remove stretch marks is by surgeries. If you find that too expensive and are looking for home remedies to make your skin stretch marks free then you need to rely on almond oil. As you have read above, almond oil has the special quality of penetrating through the skin and treating it through nutrients, and this quality is effective in removing the stretch marks as well.

Tip: Take some almond oil in your hands and then gently rub them on your stretch marks in circular motions. This will create a heated friction in your skin, which in turn will enhance blood circulation and the natural healing process. Once your stretch marks heal, your skin won't be susceptible to stretching and tearing. Plus, it will decrease the blemishes on your skin through its natural healing properties. No doubt, it is one of the easiest ways to remove stretch marks but it requires consistency and regular application.

Strengthens Nervous System

Almonds have always been associated with high brain functioning so it may come as no surprise to you that almond oil is beneficial for the nervous system as well. Its regular consumption has the power to enhance the functioning of the brain and retain memory. People who take almonds regularly can reduce the chances of amnesia in old age.

Tip: Mix one teaspoon of almond oil in a glass of milk and take it regularly. The combination of mono-saturated fats and omega-3 fatty acids is the perfect boost for brain functioning.

If you are lactose intolerant you can prepare another mixture by combining one tablespoon of Dijon mustard, vinegar and maple syrup each with three tablespoons of almond oil. Store it in a bottle and take it once a day to make your nervous system strong.

Makes Bones Strong

Massaging with almond oil is known to do miracles for bones, especially in children. Since their body is in the development phase and massaging regularly with almond oil increases blood circulation and strengthen bones and muscles. Moreover, this nutrient-rich oil is good for the skin as well. You will see that your baby's skin has turned soft, smooth and almond oil has a pleasant smell making it the ideal massage oil.

Besides babies elder people can benefit too with this oil. It is an excellent pain reliever. The high quantity of lime and calcium present in this oil can provide immediate relief from joint pain and prevent you from turning into a patient of osteoporosis. Women, in particular, should make a habit of massaging with almond oil to reduce the pain problems in the menopause stage.

If you are suffering from extreme joint pain then heat the oil a little before applying it on the skin. This will enhance its healing effects; plus, the warmth of the oil is very soothing.

Relieves Muscle Pain

The anti inflammatory and analgesic properties of almond oil can be very helpful in treating pain caused due to strained muscles. Heat some oil and apply it on the painful area, whether its neck or knee, massage it with soft and firm hands and after a few days you will feel that the pain is deteriorating. The only condition is that you need to apply it regularly.

Tip: Place two tablespoons of grounded ginger and two cups of almond oil in a slow cooker and heat it continuously for 6 hours. This will combine the extract of ginger with the nutritious almond oil. When its done transfer this warm oil to a bottle via cheesecloth, this will leave all the ginger pieces behind and you will get clear, transparent oil. Add three tablespoons of eucalyptus essential oil in the bottle stir it and place the lid.

Massage your painful muscles using this oil mixture daily and you will feel pain relieved in no time!

Anti Inflammation

If you want a cost effective wound healer then almond oil is the easiest solution available for you! Its anti-inflammatory properties are acquired from zinc which heals minor wounds, bruises and other injuries in almost no time. Moreover, the presence of monosaturated fats in this oil elevates healthy cell membranes in the skin, which means that the skin healing process fastens up.

Almond oil's anti-inflammatory properties are very effective in treating minor skin ailments like eczema, dry skin, itchiness and psoriasis as well. It hydrates skin and protects it against these common skin problems.

Tip: Combine 3 teaspoons of almond oil with 3 teaspoons of carrot seed oil and 6 to 7 drops of peppermint oil and store it in a bottle. Applying this mixture on bruises, wounds or dry skin will protect your skin from the harshness of weather and other microorganisms that damage skin.

Other Benefits

Soaps and Cosmetics Creation

Several cosmetics and soaps use almond oil as a moisturizing agent. It balances the moisture of the skin and protects it against dryness. Its presence in soaps indicates that it will make good leather; plus, it isn't harmful for the skin like other chemical based products. Similarly, almond oil in cosmetics not only retains moisture but add a sweet fragrance too.

Massage Therapies

As we have mentioned before almond oil is excellent massage oil, this is why it is used in various salons for massage and aroma therapies. It is full of nutrients, keeps the skin hydrated and enhances the blood circulation. In aromatherapy it is used as carrier oil in combination with essential oils. Almond oil's skin friendly nature makes it the best carrier oil!

Culinary Uses

Almond oil is a healthy and vitamin rich substitute for cooking oils. People who have high cholesterol levels are advised by doctors to use this oil as it has the tendency to increase the amount of good bacteria in the stomach, which in turn improves the digestive system. In addition to that, dietitians categorize this oil as healthy oil and recommend it to people who are trying to lose weight.

Here are some of the most common and popular recipes that use almond oil:

Almond Butter

Serving Size

Makes 16 servings

Cooking Time

Preparation time: 10 minutes

Cooking time: 10 minutes

Ingredients

Almond oil – 2 tsp

Toasted almonds – 1 cup

Preparation Method

1. After toasting the almonds transfer them to the food processor. Pulse them until they turn into fine powder.

2. You will see that some of the powdered almond has turned into balls, pour almond oil in the food processor and pulse once again.

3. Scrape powdered almond from the sides of the bowl and add more almond oil if required then pulse again.

4. Transfer the paste to an airtight container and store in the refrigerator.

Nutritional Facts

Calories – 25

Carbs – 1.8 g

Fat – 2.5 g

Cholesterol – 0 mg

Almond Oil with Peppermint

Serving Size

Makes 2 servings

Cooking Time

Preparation time: 1 minute

Cooking time: 3 minutes

Ingredients

Peppermint extract – Half tsp

Almond oil – Half cup

Preparation Method

1. Take out almond oil in a sauce pan and add peppermint extract in it.

2. Heat it at low heat for 3 minutes and it will start releasing its peppery fragrance.

3. Store it in a jar at room temperature.

Nutritional Facts

Calories – 484.4

Carbs – 0.1 g

Fat – 54.5 g

Cholesterol – 0 mg

Sweet and Spicy Almonds

Serving Size

Makes 4 servings

Cooking Time

Preparation time: 10 minutes

Baking time: 30 minutes

Ingredients

Almonds (unblanched) – 2 cups

Red pepper flakes (crushed) – Quarter tsp

Chili powder – Half tsp

Garlic salt – Half tsp

Cayenne pepper – 1 tsp

Almond oil – 2 tbsp

Sugar – Quarter cup

Preparation Method

1. Combine all the ingredients in a bowl except almonds.

2. Mix them properly, and when you are done mixing add almonds in the bowl.

3. Toss them around so that they are properly covered with the bowl mixture.

4. Take a baking dish and spread almonds it. Make sure that they don't overlap.

5. Heat the oven at 250°F and keep the baking dish inside the oven.

6. After 20 minutes check on the almonds. Stir them and then keep them back in the oven.

7. After 10 minutes take them out, let them cool for a while and then transfer them to an airtight jar. Store the jar in the refrigerator.

Nutritional Facts

Calories – 280

Carbs – 20 g

Fat – 21 g

Cholesterol – 0 mg

Almond Rusks

Serving Size

Makes 24 rusks

Cooking Time

Preparation time: 20 minutes

Cooking time: 45 minutes

Ingredients

Salt – 1 tsp

Baking powder – 1 ½ tsp

Almonds (finely chopped) – 1 cup

All purpose flour – 3 ½ cups

Almond oil – 1 cup

Eggs – 3

Preparation Method

1. Whisk all 3 eggs in a bowl and then add oil and sugar in it. Mix it well.

2. Now one by one start adding all the powdered ingredients in the egg. Don't forget to stir constantly or the mixture will turn into small balls. You will notice that the mixture has gained consistency and is turning into thick dough.

3. Divide that dough into 3 equal portions and then flatten each portion in a rectangular shape and place it on a greased baking dish.

4. Set the oven at 350°F and keep your baking dish in it. After 15 to 20 minutes check on it. Don't let it burn!

5. If it has taken rusk-like consistency, then take it out and let it cool before enjoying!

Nutritional Facts

Calories – 219

Carbs – 23 g

Fat – 13 g

Cholesterol – 27 mg

Chocolate Flavored Almond Butter

Serving Size

Makes 4 servings

Cooking Time

Preparation time: 5 minutes

Cooking time: 15 minutes

Ingredients

Sea salt – 1 tsp

Cocoa powder – 1 tbsp

Cherries (dried) – Quarter cup

Almond oil – 2 tbsp

Almonds – 1 cup

Preparation Method

1. Pulse almonds in the food processor. When they have turned into fine powder add all the remaining ingredients too.
2. Pulse them once again until you get a thick paste.
3. After that transfer it to a jar and store it in the refrigerator.

Nutritional Facts

Calories – 150

Carbs – 5 g

Fat – 14 g

Cholesterol – 0 mg

Nut Green Salad

Serving Size

Makes 4 servings

Cooking Time

Preparation time: 15 minutes

Cooking time: 0 minutes

Ingredients

Coarse salt – A pinch

Lemon juice (fresh) – 1 tbsp

Almond oil – 3 tbsp

Toasted almonds – Quarter cup

Golden raisins – 2/3 cup

Cilantro leaves – 2 cups

Celery stalks – 6

Preparation Method

1. Chop celery stalks and cilantro leaves.
2. Pulse almonds and raisins in the food processor until you get thick pieces.
3. Combine these four ingredients in a bowl.
4. Top it with almond oil and lemon juice.

5. Mix all the ingredients and refrigerate it for an hour before serving.

Nutritional Facts

Calories – 180

Carbs – 19 g

Fat – 12 g

Cholesterol – 0 mg

Ketchup

Serving Size

Makes 1 serving

Cooking Time

Preparation time: 5 minutes

Cooking time: 10 minutes

Ingredients

Pepper – Quarter tsp

Kosher salt – Quarter tsp

Almond oil – 1 tbsp

Peppers (jarred roasted piquillo) – Half cup

Tomato sauce – Quarter cup

Preparation Method

1. Combine all the ingredients in a food processor.

2. Pulse them until you get a thick paste-like mixture.

3. Transfer it to a jar and store it in the refrigerator.

Nutritional Facts

Calories – 310

Carbs – 48 g

Fat – 15 g

Cholesterol – 0 mg

Almond and Parsley Pesto

Serving Size

Makes 1 serving

Cooking Time

Preparation time: 5 minutes

Cooking time: 30 minutes

Ingredients

Low salt chicken broth – Quarter cup

Parmesan (grated) – Quarter cup

Almond oil – Quarter cup

Garlic cloves – 2

Thyme leaves – 1 tbsp

Toasted almonds – 1/3 cup

Parsley leaves – 1 cup

Preparation Method

1. Chop parsley leaves and place them in the food processor along with rest of the dry ingredients.

2. After that add oil and parmesan cheese and pulse once again.

3. Add salt and pepper according to your taste and take it out in a jar or glass container.

4. You can store it in refrigerate for up to few weeks.

Nutritional Facts

Calories – 720

Carbs – 11 g

Fat – 71 g

Cholesterol – 20 mg

Garlic Sauce

Serving Size

Makes 8 servings

Cooking Time

Preparation time: 15 minutes

Cooking time: 0 minutes

Ingredients

Tomatoes (diced) – 14 ½ ounces

Black pepper – Half tsp

Salt – 1 tsp

Almond oil – Quarter cup

Parsley (minced) – 2 tsp

Basil leaves – 5

Garlic cloves – 7

Almonds – Half cup

Preparation Method

1. Pulse almonds in the food processor.

2. When they have turned into fine powder, add the remaining ingredients too and pulse once again.

3. You will get a thick sauce. Take it out in a bowl and serve!

Nutritional Facts

Calories – 720

Carbs – 11 g

Fat – 71 g

Cholesterol – 20 mg

Conclusion

You must have noticed that almond oil is beneficial for all areas of life. It contains rich assortment of all the healthy minerals and vitamins that are essential for the proper growth of a body. You can greatly benefit from this oil's regular use.

So, are you ready to make transition to a healthy lifestyle?